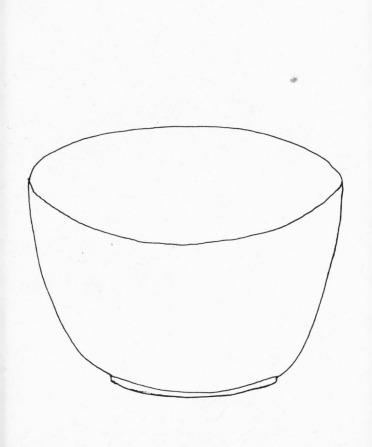

a simple concept
for controlling body weight

ONE BOWL

Don Gerrard

illustrated by Anne Kent Rush

A Random House-Bookworks Book

Copyright © 1974 by Don Gerrard

First printing, January 1974, 25,000 in paperback
                                1,500 in cloth

Typing by Jean G. Porter
Cover and Illustrations by Anne Kent Rush
Typesetting by Vera Allen Composition Service, Hayward, Ca.
   (special thanks to Irene and Rosemay)
Printed and bound under the supervision of Dean Ragland,
   Random House

This book is co-published by Random House, Inc.
                              201 East 50th St.
                              New York, N.Y. 10022

                    and   The Bookworks
                              1409 Fifth St.
                              Berkeley, Calif. 94710

Distributed in the United States by Random House, and simultaneously published in Canada by Random House of Canada Limited, Toronto.
Grateful acknowledgment is made to The National Enquirer for permission to reprint a small excerpt from Vol. 48, No. 2, September 9, 1973. Copyright © 1973 by The National Enquirer, Lantana, Florida.
Library of Congress Cataloging in Publication Data

Gerrard, Don.
One bowl.

"A Random House/Bookworks book."
1. Reducing diets.   2. Nutrition.   I. Title.
RM222.2.G47   613.2'5   73-20587
ISBN 0-394-49285-4
ISBN 0-394-70690-0 (pbk.)

Manufactured in the U.S.A.

CONTENTS

RECOMMENDED BOOKS

The Psychologist's Eat-Anything Diet, Leonard and Lillian Pearson, Wyden, 1973.

The Tooth Trip, Thomas McGuire D.D.S., Random House—Bookworks, 1972.

Getting Clear, Body Work for Women, Anne Kent Rush, Random House—Bookworks, 1973.

The Well Body Book, Mike Samuels M.D. and Hal Bennett, Random House—Bookworks, 1973.

Tassajara Cooking, Edward Espe Brown, Shambhala Publications, 1973.

Breathe Away Your Tension, Bruno H. Geba, Random House—Bookworks, 1973.

Purity of Heart Is To Will One Thing, Soren Kierkgaard, Harper & Row, 1948.

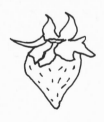

Thanks for editorial help to

Hal Bennett
Eugenia Gerrard

and especially to
Anne Kent Rush
✩

IS THIS BOOK FOR YOU?

I have written this small book as a way to share my diet discoveries with you; I am able to lose weight at any time without going hungry and without placing restrictions on the kinds of foods I eat. I do not have to think about calories, about the nutritional values of food or about eating the proper nutritional balances. I set no controls whatever on the food available to me in the world. I can eat any food that I really want. Yet I automatically control my body weight while eating in a nourishing and satisfying way.

In order to accomplish these things I pay attention to the sensation of hunger inside me each time it occurs. This familiar sensation is the first note of a whole symphony of inner sensations connected to one's natural digestive processes. They occur ceaselessly throughout every meal. I have discovered that if I see these sensations as signals from my body telling me something about the food I am eating, I can learn from them how to lose weight.

Expressed another way, *you gain weight because your head makes food decisions that ignore what your body wants.* You may not believe that your body can know what it needs or could express these needs to you as wants. You may try to follow diet systems that set their standards by the needs of an "idealized" or of an "average" body instead of your own particular body. The food recommendations that emerge are arbitrary restrictions which leave you feeling unsatisfied and sometimes punished. The result can be a hopeless conflict between foods you want to eat and a body that grows too large.

In this book I discuss ways to make contact with the digestive sensations and feelings in your body and show how to understand what they mean. You can use this knowledge to lose up to twenty pounds in about eight weeks, as I did. Since I do not know anyone who has lost more than twenty-five pounds following this diet concept I suggest you limit your expectations to that figure. Once you begin eating as I describe, you will notice changes in the way you feel within three days and will be losing weight within ten.

I also discuss 'how' you can properly establish the *range* of your normal body weight, which will vary from day to day and week to week according to your metabolism, your energy expenditure and your emotional well-being. *Since this diet concept follows natural body processes, it will lead you to your natural weight range* in several months, during which time you will lose all excess weight. If you have some image or idea of a weight or size you'd like to be different from this — perhaps smaller — you are in a position of working against natural processes trying to achieve those results.

People with chronic minor digestive complaints, like bad teeth, heartburn, acid stomach, bad breath, stomach aches, or diarrhea, can use this book to begin to understand and control their symptoms in a new way. People who regularly accompany eating or digestion with a chemical aid may discover how to end this dependency.

If these claims sound wonderful, miraculous or ridiculous to you, then your feelings mirror the fact that you don't believe in or understand the powers inherent in your own body. This is not surprising, since such knowledge is actively discouraged in our culture. Nowhere are we taught that our bodies can regulate themselves, or heal themselves. And we are not taught that our inner feelings and sensations are the signals by which this regulation or this healing is effected. On the contrary, we have been taught to ignore these *inner* signals, which come from ourselves, in favor of listening to various *outer* authorities, experts and specialists. People who try to develop a trust in their inner feelings are in a position of having to work against forces in our culture in order to achieve health. They have to overrule authority with common sense and cultural patterns with new knowledge. You are the primary source; your body is the living experience. Trust it, go with it.

I experience my life's existence on three levels

simultaneously: a cortical level (I think and reflect); a hormonal level (I feel and experience); a molecular level (I pulsate and move). However, our language lacks the words by which I can say *me* in a way that you know I mean all three levels of me at once. Instead, I must say *me* and then say *my body* or *my feelings*, as though these parts of me were not also me. The English language perpetuates a mind/body split I do not experience. Therefore, in this book when I say *me, my body, you, your body*, I am always referring to the whole person.

Our language has no singular ungendered pronoun forms. In order to avoid the clumsy expressions *he or she, him or her* throughout the book I adopt *they, them* and *their* wherever the singular pronoun should be used.

THE CONCEPT

My experience is that "food" is both a substance I eat and a group of ideas intimately connected to my ways of being in the world. These ideas form the boundaries of my personality, expressing who I am, what I want in life and how I try to get it. Since eating is one way I make my being grow, I cannot eat without experiencing many strong feelings, consciously or unconsciously, about myself, about what I am eating and about the environment and conditions under which I eat.

When and how often I feel hungry, what I choose to eat and how my body uses the food — all are expressions of my individual self.

I eat because I am hungry but I also eat to affirm my being, my personality, my sense of life. Naturally then eating is an important emotional experience. Each bite of food initiates dozens of tiny normal reactions in every part of my body, including and especially concentrated on my digestive system. From my lips to my intestines I experience fluid secretions, sensations of motion and weight, feelings of pleasure and, below my direct perception, chemical adjustments and increased molecular activity. These changes seem to me as complex as a symphony, with many individual body parts working together to make harmonious music.

This same food symphony goes on within you too, though you may have been too busy to notice it. *My diet concept begins by isolating you from external noise so that you can concentrate on your internal sounds.* Then it shows you how to interpret and evaluate these sounds for the important signals they are.

I used to eat mostly with my head, paying attention to my ideas and memories of food and to its taste, but ignoring the food once it was swallowed. Now I eat more with my whole body, in that I focus attention on how well my body can assimilate the food it receives. I try to eat foods it digests well. I call eating with my head *social eating*

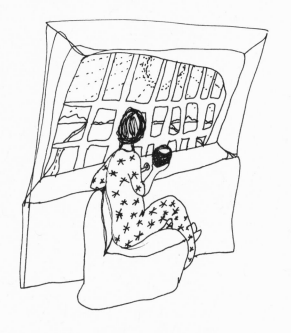

since my attention at these times is focused outside
myself; I don't know what my body feels about
the food. On the other hand, *whole body eating*
begins when I first feel hungry and ends only when
digestion is complete. It includes social eating
demands in all food considerations, but it includes
other body demands as well.

The more you eat foods you like that your
body also likes, the more harmoniously and completely your body can use them, leaving less to be
stored as fat. The more you are aware of the signals

of hunger, and of hunger ceasing, the less you will tend to overeat. Though I do not know why, these internal signals are easy to follow once you understand them. You will actually experience more pleasure when you follow them than when you don't. Over a period of time, you will see that different foods, eaten at different times of day produce different effects on your body. These effects vary according to the mood you're in, but eating too has the power to change your mood. When you strive to eat foods that are harmonious with your body signals, the best internal music is made. In other words, then your body can most efficiently use the food (no matter what food it is) and your mood will either remain good or grow better.

If you decide to follow this diet concept you will gradually *change your eating habits so that the food you eat will be more harmonious with your body.* You will modify your present diet, but perhaps not greatly. These changes can be made as gradually as you wish. Since they are dependent on the signals you receive from inside yourself, and on your interpretation of them, you will always be in complete control of your diet, which will move along according to your pleasure. Once you can experience that you really have control over your body weight, how much 'pep' or energy you have and your mood, through the food you eat, your sense of contentment, personal power and well-being will rise considerably. You will be able to move your body weight to its natural level and still please all your other (emotional) requirements about food. This book is about food attitudes; it says that as your attitudes toward food change, so will your body weight.

CHOOSE A BOWL

The first changes you make to go on this diet are not in the foods you eat. Instead, they focus on your eating patterns — that set of habits you have developed which determines *how rather than what you eat*. These changes will allow you to see the food you eat in a new way. Unless you give them a try, you will not be able to use this diet concept with much effectiveness. So, consider that you are taking a little food adventure with me, and see what may come about.

Begin by choosing a bowl that you would like to eat from. Choose a bowl that pleases you in the way it looks and feels. The bowl that I began this diet with was rather small — about three and one-half inches at the mouth, tapering to a one and one-half inch base. However, I now use a bowl almost six inches wide at the mouth. Though shape and size are flexible, your bowl should comfortably be able to hold about one cup of food.

If you can find a suitable bowl around the house, fine; if not, definitely go out and buy one. Consider antique bowls, bowls from romantic places, contemporary ceramic ones and children's bowls. I have one of each. It is important that you choose a bowl you like, that pleases you visually and feels good to hold. This is the first step.

If you think about it, *eating is a process of possession, of incorporating a part of the world into yourself,* of taking that which is not you and admitting it within your boundaries. Your bowl becomes the gateway to this process. When you put food into your bowl, you are making it your possession and preparing it for inner transformation. Every culture has rituals that acknowledge the significance of this event, including elaborate and careful washing of face and hands before eating (the Middle East), traditional forms for food preparation (the Orient), and the act of saying grace (European and American). These customs are examples of an attitude that gives spiritual significance to the intake of food. Food feeds the soul as well as the body.

Eating is a sacred act, bringing energy to sustain your life. In a sense, you could say that your life derives from one bowl.

The bowl that you have chosen to eat from is a symbol, then, for that spiritual bowl which accompanies the essence and meaning of your life. *Your bowl symbolizes your right to eat, to renew your life.* The more I eat from my bowl, the more I feel the power of this simple truth.

Once you have chosen a bowl, and feel ready to use it, begin in this way: use the bowl at every

9

meal just the way you have always used a plate. You may have difficulties at first. Certain foods do not fit easily into the bowl — a sandwich for instance. This may make you feel foolish. Also, the bowl does not allow you to keep different foods in your possession from falling together and getting mixed into each other the way a plate does. Further, your bowl will simply not hold even half as much food as a plate can. You will be forced to have less food in your possession at any one time. The answer to these dilemmas is to accept the fact that there is less food in your bowl, relax, and feel free to have "seconds" and "thirds."

I often have noticed that when people sit down to eat they regard the food on the table before them as a gift, of which they are certain to get a share. This is as it should be. One is used to surveying their full plate, or a table of food, and immediately sensing how the food is their possession, theirs to own and enjoy. The look in a person's face at such moments is definitely the look of receiving a gift — the expectation, the anticipation of a new possession. Can you feel this in yourself?

What's going to happen to your sense of possession when all you have before you is one small bowl of food? One solution is to expand and redirect your sense of possession. Let it cover the entire table of food before you. If you are eating with people who use plates, their sense of possession will be more confined to their plates than yours to your bowl; yours can range over all the 'free' food on the table. I will show you how I extend my sense of food possession much further than the table in the section called HUNTING.

EAT IN COURSES

When you feel comfortable with the bowl you've selected, begin to eat from it every meal you eat at home. However, try to alter your current diet as little as possible, eating just the same foods as always, but adapting them to bowl eating.

The simplest way to solve the problems caused by your bowl's small size is to put only one food in it at a time. In other words, eat in courses. If you previously ate three to five different foods at a meal, then fill your bowl three to five times in succession, each fill being a different food. You will find that it takes you a bit longer to eat this way, but you become increasingly aware of the taste of each food. Notice that you have the option of washing your bowl between each fill. You may observe right away how different your eating rhythm is from family or friends who eat beside you from plates.

Try to make yourself comfortable eating this way — from your bowl, in courses — before you move on to develop this diet concept further. For example, it takes time to figure out how to eat a breakfast of cereal, eggs, sausage and toast all from a bowl. It takes time for it to feel okay to eat foods one at a time. It also takes more time to do the eating. You will be surprised, however, just how satisfying this can be. After a meal, each food will linger more distinctly in your memory, and eating will have been a series of gifts, linked together by your bowl.

Every mealtime you will follow all your old diet habits, except for these changes: you eat from your bowl; you claim the entire table of 'free' food before you as potential food choices; you eat in courses, filling your bowl with only one food at a time. Within a few days, you should begin to feel at home with your bowl, and familiar with how you like to eat from it.

Take your time getting acquainted with this change in your eating pattern. Persons who regularly eat alone will probably adjust to bowl eating faster than those who eat with family or friends. If you do the latter, remember that you have to give these other people time to adjust to this bowl idea too.

Have you begun to wonder how you can use your bowl when eating in a restaurant or at someone's home? Don't try to. For the moment, confine your new diet concept entirely to your own living space. Later, I will talk about the special problems of 'eating out.'

EAT ALONE

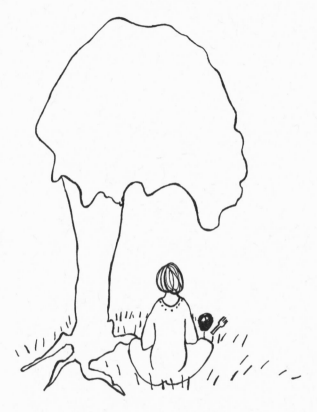

The next development in this concept is to begin eating alone. Maintain your same diet of foods as before, eating from your bowl, in courses. But now begin eating alone. Pick a favorite room or area of your living space and go there alone with your bowl. Make yourself comfortable in all the ways you know you like, and eat. Once you think about it, you might choose to eat in bed, or on your back porch, or in a corner of the living room. Help yourself. You need not always eat in the same place, but do always eat in a place you like. Do not watch television, read or otherwise distract yourself from the pleasure of eating. Put your attention on the food in your possession, relax and enjoy the sensations of its taste and of chewing and swallowing it. Eat standing, sitting or lying down – whatever pleases you. During this time, allow eating to become a luxury in your life. Bask in this luxury.

You may find this one part of my diet concept the most difficult to accept. If the idea of eating alone makes you feel uncomfortable, try to find out why. However, it is important that you carry out this part of the diet development for this reason: eating alone is the only way you can begin to become aware of the sensations of food and digestion within you. It is the only way to begin to understand this natural, inner language. When you eat with other people, your attention is on them, or on your relationship to them, rather than on the experience of eating. Also, the tempo and rhythm of your eating pattern – how fast or slow you eat – is dramatically effected when you eat while talking with others. Later, after you have become thoroughly familiar with the inner language of eating, it will be possible to eat with others and still keep part of your attention attuned to your inner experience. But for now, eat alone.

Naturally if you live with other people more adjustments must be made. If you are the person in a relationship who regularly prepares food for others, then do so, announce the meal, and take your bowl (your first course) to your chosen eating place to eat alone. If another person regularly prepares food for you, you will just take your bowl of food away to eat alone. Though at first it may not seem so, most people have less trouble establishing this routine than they expect.

If mealtimes are the only times you have together with family or friends, you may feel that you must choose between this diet and your family. However, you could arrange to eat before or after everyone else. This way you could satisfy your diet and still socialize with your family when they eat. Our family solved this problem by disbanding organized meals altogether. However, I do not recommend this step for you unless you are naturally moved to it. Everyone will find their own special way of handling this problem.

Let the idea of eating alone initiate a new food training period in your life. Let the next several months be a time apart, in which you will focus your attention on food and on how your body responds to it. Then, as you develop new attitudes toward the food you eat, you will see how to begin re-integrating eating into your social life, and you will gradually do so.

THE DE-SOCIALIZATION OF FOOD

For most people, controlling body weight is intimately connected to the socialization of food. When you begin to eat alone, you may begin to feel lonely, bored, cold, depressed or not hungry. Don't let these feelings confuse you. Once you are into your new eating pattern regularly, you will discover new pleasures to replace your old familiar ones. On the other hand, people also have felt energized, liberated, relieved or starved when beginning to eat alone on this diet. Both kinds of responses are testimony to the power of the socialization of food in a person's life. You may experience neither or you may experience both. Either way, you will find that once you are settled into the routine of eating alone, the amount and kind of food you want to eat has changed in some way. In other words, *everyone eats some foods in certain ways just because they are eating with other people.* The harder it is for you to accept eating alone, the more distinctly changed your diet is likely to become once you can do it regularly.

This part of my concept — the de-socialization of food — may be your greatest hurdle. Therefore, go slow. There are no time limits. You are eating whatever you wish but trying to make changes in the *way* you eat. You are isolating the food distractions in your life: seeking a quiet room, going in, closing the door and being with your private food feelings. This is a perfectly natural response. You may never have realized before that social eating changes your body's response to food so much. Therefore, give yourself time to see whether what I am saying is true for you. Most people, after three or four days of eating alone, find that they prefer it to social eating most of the time because of the quiet personal pleasure it brings.

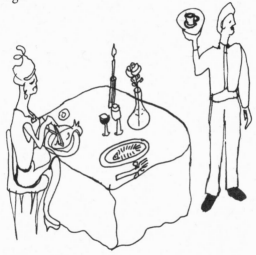

If your mate objects to this stage in your diet because when you eat alone they have to eat alone, by all means be with them when they eat. Have tea with them, but eat before or after. Share with them these diet ideas and work out a common agreement before you start. Our culture teaches and practices the socialization of food as an important part of personal life. Take the time you need to work out the problems of de-socialization you have, proceeding further only when you are comfortably eating alone and enjoying it.

THE FOOD SYMPHONY

When you have developed the diet concept this far, you will have made many changes in your former eating patterns. You now eat your normal diet of foods from a bowl, in courses, and you eat alone. You focus your attention on the food you eat – how each bite tastes and what it feels like to chew and swallow. You probably are eating less food now, just because it's easier to tell when you feel full. But you probably find eating more satisfying than before and you look forward to it as a time in which you can relax and be alone with yourself. These changes are simple to describe, but profound in their effect upon your mood.

After more than thirty years of eating, I am finally beginning to see that there is more to it than just putting food in my mouth. I now believe that eating is one of the most complex activities I undertake each day, and I am learning to treat eating with an increasingly greater respect. I see that eating begins with the very first tiny vibration of hunger inside me – a vibration that grows until I am set into motion, hunting food. I see that eating includes deciding what food I want to eat, the way I prepare it, under what circumstances I eat it, how fast or slow I chew and swallow, and the process of digestion and assimilation that goes on without my conscious direction during and after the meal. In fact, eating is not truly concluded until my body eliminates as waste the parts of the food it cannot use. All this is eating; it is like a symphony – many elements must come together in harmony. When they do, music is made and one is nourished. When they don't the result is noise and discomfort.

You will lose weight and gain energy as you learn to increase the harmony in your internal food symphony. It is a simple and natural thing to do, once you understand how to do it. In order to develop this understanding you have to create a space in your life in which to focus closely on the food you eat. Everything you have done so far in this diet brings you to this space.

FIVE PRINCIPLES

You are now ready to explore the foods you eat, to find out which ones fit your body well and which ones are discordant, creating upset (digestive upset) and waste (stored as fat). Once you can feel the sensations of discomfort or upset within you caused by eating a certain food, then you can choose whether you want to continue eating that food. On the other hand, when you can feel the sensations of harmony and energy brought to you by a food, you can choose whether you would prefer to eat foods like that one more often. The more you substitute harmonious foods for those that cause you discomfort, the more completely your body can use that food and the less it has to store as fat.

☆ *You will be able to lose weight by decreasing your consumption of disruptive foods and increasing your consumption of harmonious ones.* This first principle is the key to my diet concept. However, in order for it to be effective, you must apply it in concert with four others.

☆ *Eat whenever you are hungry,* as often as you are hungry, but stop the minute hunger ceases. This will be *before* you feel full. Often I eat six or more times a day, always from my bowl, alone. I never deprive myself of anything I want or let myself go hungry, but I always cease eating when the sensation of hunger fades.

☆ *Eat only one food each "meal."* Occasionally I will eat two foods and rarely three at a meal. Whenever I eat more than one, I do so in courses. But nine-tenths of my meals now are single course meals.

☆ *When you get hungry, make a search to find just the right food* you want to eat that moment. Recognize that different moods on different days will bring the desire for many different foods. I consider hunting food an important part of my daily life, and I give time to it, all the time I need.

☆ The same food prepared in different ways will have strikingly different effects on your digestive system. I have found, in general, that foods prepared with seasonings and spices or by mixing with other foods tend to be less harmonious than the same foods prepared plainly and eaten alone. Thus, if I really enjoy a food that is disruptive to me, I change the manner of its preparation until I have made it more harmonious. In this way *I have never had to abandon eating any food I liked.*

I did not apply these principles to my diet overnight; they evolved gradually over a period of months. I began by applying only the second and third — each time I felt hungry I considered it a "meal" and ate until I was no longer hungry. And I ate only one food for each meal. In this way I pretty much conformed to my former diet of foods, eating just about whatever my family ate.

At this time I had not met Leonard and Lillian Pearson nor heard about their food workshops, at the Pearson Institute, even though they were held in Berkeley where I live. A friend of mine did attend a workshop, and came to see me one day filled with enthusiasm. She told of spending several hours experimenting with just chewing food and how satisfying that was. She told of eating *one bean* and completely losing her sense of hunger. She told about foods that *hum* and foods that *beckon,* and how important it was to search out just the right food you want to eat every meal. For an hour she told me these amazing things. From this one conversation I was fired with new enthusiasm for food exploration and went on to complete my diet concept.

In this book I do not talk about the *psychology of food*, which could be defined as understanding and explaining why people eat as they do, because the Pearsons have pioneered this field in their book *The Psychologist's Eat-Anything Diet.* But thanks to the Pearsons, I could add the fourth principle to my ideas – to always search out the food I really wanted to eat. The last one – learning how to prepare food – developed naturally as a matter of course, and directly implemented and refined the first four.

In this stage of my diet development, I would eat from my bowl, alone, at the regular breakfast, lunch and dinner times my family had established and then also one to three more times in the day, whenever I felt hungry. You might try this as an easy way to *shift into a pattern of eating from hunger, and out of a pattern of eating from habit.*

Looking back over the five principles I have just discussed, you may feel that I have given you too much new information to absorb all at once. In practice, however, you will find these ideas simple to apply and the results direct and effective. Move into them slowly, at your own natural speed. When

I became impatient in the early days of my new eating pattern I would remind myself that I did not accumulate my extra weight in a single day, but rather over months of eating. This accumulation occurred slowly as a natural process. So did my decision to lose this extra weight. In the same way, this concept must become a natural process. Allow yourself the time it will take to adjust to these changes in your life.

LEARNING THE SIGNALS

I said earlier that the key to this diet concept lies in your ability to distinguish disruptive foods from harmonious ones, and in your decision to eat more of the latter. Once I could clearly feel a variety of sensations from the different foods I ate including which were harmonious to me and which not, deciding to eat more harmoniously was a simple matter of choice. When you have begun to eat only one food at each meal you take, and have begun to eat these meals more from hunger than from habit, you can begin to focus on your body feelings, seeking to recognize your body's response to each food you eat. Each time you go to your chosen eating spot for a meal, observe the following things:

1. Where in your body do you feel hungry? Mouth? Throat? Stomach? Just sit for a minute and feel that sensation of hunger.

You should do this each meal until your hunger sensations are thoroughly familiar to you. They will emanate from different parts of your digestive system according to your mood, whether you are working or resting, the time of day, your general health, etc., and they will not always be the same intensity or quality of sensation. Don't judge them; just feel them.

2. Look at and smell the food in your bowl. Does it seem to be just the very food you most want to eat right now? If not, put it aside and find one that promises greater satisfaction. If one part of your digestive system distinctly wants the food, which part is it? Just feel these sensations of food anticipation for a moment. Gradually, they will become very familiar to you, though of course they will vary among foods, and as your moods vary. See if over a period of days you can detect a pattern to them.

3. Now take one bite of food, and chew it thoroughly. How does it feel to your tongue, teeth, cheeks? What, if anything, is happening to your feeling of hunger as you chew? Try to focus your attention on chewing and enjoy chewing this bite of food for as long as you like.

4. Swallow the bite of food. Try to follow that bite as it settles into your stomach. If

you can't feel it going down, imagine you can feel it going down. Can you feel it in your stomach? If not, imagine that you can. For a moment just focus on the sensation of this bite of food in your stomach. During this time, has there been any change in your feeling of hunger? What does the rest of your body feel? Can you eat and also remain relaxed? (Relaxed breathing, pleasant mental activity, minimal muscular tension and comfortable posture?)

5. Repeat this simple, silent procedure for the first five bites of food each meal for several weeks. You will gain a new familiarity with the food you eat, and in addition collect valuable information about your body's inner feelings toward every food. You may find foods that suddenly do not taste so good, and others that taste better than you ever expected. You may find that the first few bites of some foods will produce a noticeable effect in your stomach, while others seem to have little effect even a half hour after eating. And you may find foods that cause digestive upset, in the form of mild pain, burping, gas, heartburn, or more severely, diarrhea.

But generally speaking, the sensations you are seeking in your body are more subtle than those commonly recognized as digestive upset. As you try to focus on what's happening to a bite of food inside of you, see whether you can feel these kinds of sensations:

emptiness
an area of emptiness
conversely, a feeling of weight, or heaviness or
    a heavy area
weight moving from one place to another
weight turning over and over
weight that flows like liquid
weight suddenly released, then emptiness

pressure
pressure building up
pressure decreasing
pressure suddenly released
pressure changing
pressure moving from one place to another
pressure changing as a result of weight changes

temperature
a food swallowed that feels warm
a food swallowed that feels cold
a body area beginning to feel warm
a body area beginning to feel cold
a body area changing temperature
temperature changes as a result of pressure
    changes
temperature changes as a result of weight
    changes

movement
a slow movement
a rhythmical, repetitive movement
a rapid, vibratory movement
a movement that grows
a movement that diminishes

a movement as a result of pressure changes
a movement as a result of weight changes
a movement as a result of temperature changes
movements of body organs
a change in intensity of movement of an organ
a muscle you tighten
a muscle you tighten as a result of changes in
    weight, pressure, temperature or movement

sound
an area of sound
a continuous, gurgling sound
a sharp, one-time sound
a sound that begins, changes or ends as a
    result of changes in any of the above
    characteristics

You will realize right away that of course you
recognize these sensations, and perhaps other
variations and combinations of them I haven't
listed. They are merely those little feelings that
always seem to be going on inside your body. Pay
attention to them. *Consider them messengers to
you, sending you signals or messages about the
food you have eaten.* You will get a signal (or more

than one) with every bite of food you take. These signals may come from your mouth area, throat, stomach or intestines — which means anywhere up and down the length of your torso. They usually begin when you first feel hunger, grow stronger and more varied when you begin to eat, continue strong for a half hour after you eat (sometimes longer) and finally conclude only after you eliminate waste. This duration — from hunger through eating to elimination — can be considered one complete food cycle. Usually you will begin several food cycles before completely concluding previous ones, so that there are always many foods in different stages of different cycles in your body sending signals all at once. It is enough for our purposes to consider just those signals that are strongest immediately before, during and for a half-hour after eating.

All of these signals are a part of your normal digestive and assimilative body processes. All of them come to you in the form of sensations or feelings, having three general patterns:

1. the strongest signals are usually more important than the weakest
2. their intensity and quality changes while you eat (over a period of time you will see a pattern to these changes)
3. *judge the meaning of each signal by how it makes you feel.*

In other words, these food sensations will definitely effect your general sense of well-being. If you have stomach pains, you feel irritable and unproductive; when you have eaten well, you feel buoyant and optimistic. Before eating you feel slightly nervous, charged, empty, weak. Afterwards you feel drowsy, relaxed, contented. A little later you are filled with energy and purpose.

Each time you eat, listen for a minute or two to all the signals you can get from one bite of food. Then, notice any changes you feel in your sense of well-being as you eat. Since you are eating only one food for your meal, you will be able to relate any changes directly to that particular food.

You are trying to evaluate the food you have just eaten; but how can you be sure if it really is harmonious to your body? I dealt with this question at first by not worrying about it too much. Some foods clearly made me feel good; others clearly did not. Still others felt okay, but I wasn't really sure about them. Unless or until I decided that a food was definitely upsetting I continued to eat it, though I tried to pay closer attention to it in the eating. Gradually, I developed three criteria to help me evaluate the meaning of the many signals I received:

1. *Every food I eat effects my mood.* The most harmonious foods either make me feel good about myself or keep me feeling good. Foods that leave me feeling worse than when I began to eat I consider not harmonious, and I avoid them.

2. *Every food I eat changes the available*

energy I have. Some foods make me feel drowzy, some sluggish, some charged up. I rate any food I eat according to whether it increases my energy or reduces it.

3. *Every food I eat effects my overall body stability.* Some foods make me feel fat. heavy, bulky, massive. Others make me feel tall, thin, lithe. Still others make me feel physically out of touch, disconnected, or unbalanced. These and many similar body sensations, though subtle, are just as real to me as my mood or my energy, and I give them equal attention.

I identify all these phenomena as intimate parts of myself, and recognize that changes occur in all of them continually. I have found that during the course of a day I can easily notice changes in my mood, my energy and my body feelings produced by the food I eat.

Though I can always feel a connection between the signals I get while eating and digesting food and the changes in mood, energy and body feelings the food produces, this connection is complex, since the possible combinations of signals and feelings are immense. Therefore it would be impossible to catalog them all. Instead, I just watch the overall patterns. If, when I eat, the food tastes good, dissipates my hunger, produces no unpleasant inner signals and does not make me feel irritated or depressed, sluggish or nervous, full or heavy, I consider that I have eaten pretty well. I have learned to look for *level foods,* foods which tend to maintain the good attitude place I am in, which keep my energy flowing steadily and which do not interrupt my sense of well-being.

BRANCHING OUT

Once you are regularly eating according to these outlines, you are no doubt already undergoing body changes. Certainly you are losing weight. Certainly eating is a more calm and meaningful experience for you. Most probably your body feels different; you have more energy, feel lighter, enjoy better moods. Take the time to appreciate these changes. Don't drive yourself too hard. Now you are confident that this diet idea works for you, so there's no hurry. Try not to hold yourself within too strict limits.

Also, branch out. Move away from the foods familiar to you and begin to try the ones you rarely eat. Many factors combine to limit the range of foods people enjoy, not the least of which are habit and convenience. Most people could easily prepare a wide selection of foods, but choose instead to eat over and over again the ones they especially like. However, you now have a whole new set of criteria to apply to foods. *You no longer judge a food just by its taste in your mouth, but by your inner body experience of it as well.*

31

New possibilities exist.

In this situation for the first time, I conducted a number of food experiments for myself, the results of which eventually carried my personal food evolution yet one step further. Here's what I did.

☆ I decided to prepare all my meals myself (or as many as I reasonably could).

☆ I began to experiment with the foods I would eat at a given time of day — trying meat or potatoes in the morning, for instance, and eggs or cereal at night. In other words, I decided to subject time-of-day foods to inner criteria and found what I suspected — that I have previously confined myself within narrow limits unnecessarily.

☆ I searched for 'new' foods to eat, ones I had rarely or never eaten before. The result of this exploration, after several months, was to widen my food vocabulary, giving greater variety in my eating experience, and more food pleasure.

☆ I began to vary my methods of food preparation. At this time I was eating from my bowl five or six times a day, alone, but I was eating within the range of my family's traditional diet of foods. I soon found that just by varying food preparation I could move into new tastes, and new possibilities of harmony in a food where formerly there was none. Though I ate only one food per meal, frequently that food was itself actually a combination of foods. Usually this combination consisted of small quantities of several foods added to one dominant one. I decided to try moving away from these combinations. I avoided eating casseroles and stews. I found that I felt better even though I could successfully eat the same foods separately.

This last experiment led me to others. I tried eliminating all cooking oils and traditional spices from my food preparation. Later, I tried eliminating all fried foods. Still other times I eliminated all forms of sugar, all caffeine, all salt and pepper, all beef or pork. Over a period of time I varied my food preparation in any way I though of or heard about that sounded good. The diet I eat now includes many foods I have used all my life, prepared more simply than before. I recount this adventure to encourage you, when you feel ready, to look at preparation as a good way to expand your food possibilities, and to consider this area of food awareness a natural part of your diet concept.

HUNTING

Each time I get those first familiar signals of hunger inside me I try to stop what I am doing and head for my hunting grounds — the kitchen.

Hunting food is an important part of the eating process to me because it is my expression of food possession. It makes me secure to know I possess a hunting ground where a selection of food is always available. I allow myself to enjoy these feelings and I often make a game of them.

Once in the kitchen I try to imagine all the different places food is stored — the refrigerator, the pantry, the cabinets, cupboards and shelves — and what food is where. Then I try to let my sense of possession extend over all these areas. "This is my hunting ground for food" I will tell myself.

Now I begin to try to match a food to my desires. I do this by handling, fondling, poking, squeezing, smelling, fantasizing and examining as many foods as it takes to find just the right one. Usually I make my selection within three or four minutes, but there have been times on occasion when I remained frustrated for up to a half hour because I couldn't settle on a food. If, at those times, I gave in to expediency and ate just any food I usually continued to be frustrated after the meal.

Take the time to declare a hunting ground in

your house and in your feelings, and use it. This idea also makes supermarket shopping more interesting.

WEIGHT

I weighed myself just at the time I was beginning to develop this diet concept but it was an accidental thing, an impulse at an airport in Hawaii. I did not weigh myself again for eight weeks, after I had lost twenty pounds. But I knew when I was losing weight and I knew approximately how much I was losing during this period. I advise you not to judge your progress on this diet from a scales. Judge it instead from your feeling about yourself. Notice changes in the way your body feels, and in your available energy. Weight loss is always accompanied by other changes because excess weight accumulation is only the end product of your eating patterns and digestive processes. *It is not the removal of weight so much as changing these processes that is your goal.* The weight loss will naturally follow.

Available Energy

I have used the word *energy* and the phrase *available energy* frequently in this book. One function of the digestive process is the production of energy for the body. However, many physical and psychological events combine to tie up this energy unproductively, or to drain it off. Therefore, I speak of available energy as a way of acknowledging the relativity of your energy supply. I assume that no matter how much energy you feel you have, you could always have more because more is potentially in the body, but unavailable for your everyday use. More harmonious use of foods will produce more energy for your use, both because the body can use the food more efficiently and because the regular accumulation of excess fat will cease. As you develop this diet concept you will feel that you have more energy, and you will feel other new body sensations. These indications of weight loss are as reliable as a scales, but they don't measure in pounds. Once you identify these sensations it will be like weighing yourself from inside.

Every morning I look myself over on the outside (in a mirror) and I feel myself on the inside. I do not have a scales. Constant use of a scales is one way to become afraid of yourself, or to punish yourself. It can lead you away from developing trust in your inner signals.

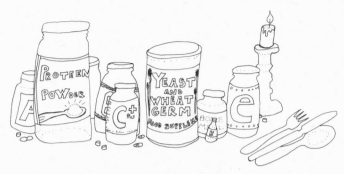

NUTRITION

Understanding nutritional needs, counting calories and developing a balanced diet were important problems for our parents, and are standards tools for describing body metabolism. But if your parents did their homework you have an intuitive understanding of these concepts that will be adequate to your basic health care. It's the scientists and the researchers who need to talk about the digestive process as objective phenomena. You don't have to, *you can live your body metabolism.*

I believe that when your body really wants a food, it can efficiently use that food, no matter the caloric content or low nutritional level that food would measure in the laboratory. It has been demonstrated that what you feel about yourself when you eat can change the nutritional meaning of any food in your body. I believe that when you crave a food, you should definitely eat it; I see cravings as authentic body signals. Most cravings are not sugar-oriented, but in our culture it's only the sugar ones that people allow themselves to satisfy. The Pearsons, in their book, *The Psychologist's Eat-Anything Diet*, clearly show you how to distinguish true cravings from idea foods that feed only your mouth or your image.

Dr. Linus Pauling, participating with five other nutritional experts in a panel discussion in Arizona in 1973 on popular misconceptions about nutrition, had this to say about the validity of the 'balanced diet.' "The balanced diets publicized nowadays may not meet the needs of one person in a thousand." And he added, "People shouldn't rely on the minimum daily requirement standards set for vitamins and minerals." Dr. Roger Williams, a biochemist at the University of Texas added, "Nutritional needs vary with every individual. Too little is known about these variations to decide what is a balanced diet and for whom." Dr. Pauling responded to the question whether a certain food or vitamin can be good for one condition and bad for another. "I've heard it said that Vitamin C might be good for colds but bad for kidneys. This is ridiculous. Any nutrient that is good for one part of the body will benefit the entire body."*

These men are remarkable for their openness. My experience is that most doctors condemn anything that hasn't been measured in the

* *National Enquirer*, Vol. 48, No. 2, September 9, 1973.

laboratory. They forget that the laboratory was devised over many centuries as a tool for studying human beings, but that *the primary source*, the reality, *lies in the human*, not the laboratory. Learn to trust your inner signals. You are the primary source. Your body events are your reality.

LIQUIDS

Think about the liquids you drink in a day. How many are there? Coffee, beer, water, tea, soft drinks, liquor, orange juice. It's a long list. All of them I consider foods, and I treat them as foods. Once I regularly ate one food per meal, from my bowl, alone, I refrained from drinking with the meal. Then, when I wanted something to drink, that drink was a food which I subjected to ONE BOWL criteria — I drank, alone, one swallow at a time, listening for inner signals about this food.

If you doubt that the common liquids you drink act in your digestive system as foods, experiment for yourself. For one week eat according to the ONE BOWL concept but drink freely at all your meals. Then, for the next week, consider everything you drink a meal. Do not drink as you eat and subject your drinking to ONE BOWL criteria. When you feel thirsty, hunt for just the right drink you want. As you drink, listen to your inner signals. I find that eating one food and drinking one food together at a meal has the same effect as eating two foods that meal: the signals from one food blur signals from the other.

But don't foods you drink digest much faster than foods you eat? They seem to. But different foods I eat digest at different rates anyway. I see liquid and solid foods all on a continuum; some digest faster than others, but they all vary tremendously in the range of their many effects on me.

SNACKS

As I evolved this diet concept I realized that the distinction between meals and 'snacks' had been completely lost. My snacks were my meals. Any food could be eaten at any time in any quantity I really wanted. No longer were my meals obligations and my snacks fun, a divisive concept that has allowed food companies to make fortunes. Now all foods could be fun, or none of them. I regained control of everything.

No longer did I worry whether eating this food now would ruin my appetite later. Of course it would! One effect of eating is to ruin your appetite. Now I could eat chocolate cake all day long if I really wanted it. The guilt was gone.

I experienced a tremendous elation when the impact of this discovery hit me. Every meal a snack! Now, I regularly subject fun foods to ONE BOWL criteria and decide for myself whether they really are fun.

EATING OUT

I have never attempted to eat from my bowl in public, either at a restaurant or at someone's home. My bowl is a personal possession, and an intimate part of my private eating space. But restaurant eating is almost unavoidable in our society, so I have had to make my peace with it while remaining true to my diet needs.

Restaurants almost always serve too large portions and food is highly socialized there. It is hard to hear my body over all the noise. These things lead me to conclude that restaurant eating means over-eating, and I just go with that. I accept these things as a real part of eating out. I am not afraid of restaurant eating anymore; it has lost much of its power over me. On the other hand, now that I eat more with my whole body, I see that there is always better food at home. Restaurant eating is sugary eating. I come away from it nervous not relaxed, socially stimulated but physically upset, often with symptoms of minor indigestion. Taken altogether, I avoid restaurants when I can.

When I can't, I try to pick from the menu carefully, visualizing each food listed and asking myself whether I really want that food. The Pearsons recommend that you choose what you want to eat before opening the menu. I visualize my bowl as I eat, trying to measure how much a bowlful of food would be. When hunger ceases, I try to leave food on the plate. But this is hard to do, since all the social conventions are insulted. Restaurant eating is an unpleasant experience.

One inescapable conclusion lies before me: the social food conventions in our culture are *unhealthy*. They lead me away from myself, they make my deny myself. I, in turn, try to avoid situations in which they can get at me.

Eating at someone else's home is a little better. I have more control because I am freer to pick and choose among the food. And frequently I can tell the people beforehand about my diet. I do not say "I am on a diet," but rather, "Since I have been following this food concept I feel better." This approach usually prevents my getting into that spot where I have to choose between overeating and hurting someone's feelings. Also, invariably someone at the table turns out to be very interested in new food and diet ideas, and usually a good food conversation results.

People on diets often feel guilty, as if being overweight was evil, and dieting was a distasteful way of making retribution. They feel guilty no matter which way they go; the result is they have no power over food in their life, and cannot really enjoy eating. I avoid this dilemma by making my diet concept a philosophy of life, something I am proud of. Now I find that many, many other people will talk about the meaning of food in their lives because they see they can talk to me without guilt. Try this approach with your friends. It may make eating out more meaningful.

Carry Food With You

I have learned one thing further. I carry food with me all the time I am away from my living space! I know that every two or three hours I must eat to keep my energy flow level, so I stay prepared for that. When I attend business conferences I either find a time when it's all right to eat the food I've brought or I excuse myself and go eat it privately. There is no reason to ignore body signals of hunger just because you are in a social situation. Use your creativity to make a good food space for yourself.

Once I had learned how to understand my inner food signals I found that they operated every day regardless of social customs. In order to make this diet concept work, I found that I had to follow it regularly. But more profoundly, I found that I *wanted* to follow it regularly. I soon preferred feeling good and having a steady energy flow through the day to the old, erratic sensations and confusions I had always experienced. This made it really important to me to stay with my inner food feelings, no matter the social situation.

I believe a similar experience will happen for you. When it does, you will find ways to circumvent the barriers social situations create against maintaining your chosen food habits.

FOOD PREPARATION

Most people in our culture eat food prepared by another person most of their lives. This practice is a more subtle form of food socialization than eating with other people is, since it means you eat food dominated by the mood and the taste of another person. Or worse still, that person tries to please you, to anticipate the taste you would like, so that the food fits no one's mood really. The result is that we all silently agree to like a certain narrow range or selection of food preparations. This is the process by which families build up their eating patterns. It's also the process you are trying to break free of by eating alone.

I finally realized I could do this only by preparing all my own food as frequently as possible. Once I began to do so, a new world opened before me, and food preparation, preceded by hunting, became a new life adventure.

The most important ingredient in food preparation is my mood. I like to be hungry but in a carefree state, physically and emotionally relaxed, when I begin to prepare my food. If I have chosen it well, getting just the right food to eat, I want to prepare it lovingly and creatively. Usually I imagine first how I will prepare it. This mental projection can be just an instant flash or can take several moments of elaborate decision, and it allows me to test out what I want to do with my food before eating it. Sometimes I want to dream or fantasize about it; sometimes I want to caress or fondle it. Sometimes I play with it. Sometimes I conquer it. Occasionally, I am just efficient and business-like in my preparation of it. All of these moods and many more are a necessary part of eating to me now. When I allow myself to express my mood in food preparation it whets my appetite and also satisfies something deep within me.

In such a mood state I really look at the food and really touch it. I wash it and cut it while I think about washing it and cutting it. My attention really is on the food because I really am interested in it. Usually by the time I am ready to eat it I know it pretty well. Food preparation means preparing the food and myself for the coming transformation we both will undergo in eating. This food I hold in my hands will soon be a part of me. I have to get myself ready for that.

Seasonings

I have learned to season my foods with small amounts of other foods — which is what commercial seasonings are anyway, but mine are fresh. Among my favorite seasonings I use celery, pecans, walnuts, cheese, mushrooms, parsley, olives, radishes. Each of these seasonings was subjected to ONE BOWL criteria; each evolved over a period of months. Like the foods I eat, the seasonings I use slowly change as I grow and change.

Tassajara Cooking

I have found and begun to use a new book to strengthen my imaginary food preparations. It's called *Tassajara Cooking* and devotes its attention to many foods by focusing on one food each in turn. It showed me how to get to know a food as I prepared it and gave me many new preparation ideas. It has no regular recipes to follow but helped me invent some for myself. It sometimes advocates mixing foods together for a meal. I just skip that part. I found that by reading it like a story I could take many imaginary food preparation adventures.

FURTHER BODY DEVELOPMENT

Going further physically means expanding the attention you focus on your digestive system to include your mouth and teeth, and your bowels. If you find that getting in touch with your body functions through the concepts presented here is meaningful to you, then you may be interested in trying these further explorations.

Teeth

The way I explore is simplicity itself. I am interested in learning what my teeth feel like before and after I eat, and in how my bowels function to excrete waste. Both teeth and bowels are taboo areas in our culture; both are areas of our bodies about which we all have strong unspoken feelings. I am convinced that self-knowledge and body health go together, so I decided to explore these taboo places.

If I try to describe what my teeth feel like, I find it difficult to do. But after brushing them well, then flossing them, I know they feel different than before. After a meal I sit for a minute and feel my teeth. They definitely are different now, a new feeling. Anytime I run my tongue over them I can feel where there are food-covered surfaces and little patches of food. Eating different foods leaves me with different tooth-surface sensations.

Gradually over a year I found I preferred the way my teeth felt when clean. So after I eat, I usually do this. First I run my tongue over all the surfaces, cleaning off the food. Then I use water to rinse my mouth. These things I can do even when eating out. At the first chance I brush. I find it easy to carry a toothbrush everywhere I go. In public, there's always a restroom.

I learned from Dr. Thomas McGuire's *The Tooth Trip* how to brush and floss to prevent cavities. I learned to tell by the feel of my tongue and the taste in my mouth when my teeth were dirty. I learned to brush part of the time without toothpaste because its taste confuses my ability to tell when my teeth really are clean. I also learned from this book that contrary to a lot of expensive advertising bad breath is caused by poor eating and digestive habits. Adopting ONE BOWL criteria allowed me to give up mouthwash. I have been exploring food in my life for two years now. An excellent primer on food and diet in *The Tooth Trip* got me started.

Elimination

I understand the basic movement of biological

life to be a two-part process. The body gathers to itself new possessions and eliminates from itself used materials. This movement has been described as charge and discharge and as transposition, but however you view it, it is the basic biological rhythm. Our culture has been characterized as one in which people easily add possessions, but give them up only with difficulty. This possessive trait may explain why we consider elimination and the organs of elimination taboo. I sometimes get the image of people grown fat because they eat but don't eliminate. They prefer to store food up within themselves rather than surrender it back to the world.

My point is that elimination is just as important to the organism as eating. I have explored my feelings about elimination in this way. Each morning I lay on the floor, with my knees up and the bottoms of my feet flat on the floor. I tried to focus my attention on my intestines just inside my anus and I waited to feel movement there. For many mornings nothing happened. Sometimes I imagined I felt the movement. Sometimes I grew very angry with myself for wasting time in this way.

When I actually defecated, I would never push. My plan was to get in touch with the natural intestinal movements in my body and to see whether I could control them.

After almost a year at this work I have made progress in contacting this inner movement. I have found that changes in my diet, through ONE BOWL criteria, have resulted in a new, freer elimination pattern that gives me added assurance about the health of my digestive system. I have found that elimination never requires pushing or straining and that it is an important body function to me, one to which I want to give my attention. I definitely spend less time and energy worrying about this function now and I feel that the work I have done has been well repaid.

The only book I know that could help you explore your elimination processes is Dr. Bruno Geba's *Breathe Away Your Tension*. From this book I learned how to relax any one part of my body and how to focus my attention on the sensations of feeling there. The book is also useful to persons with chronic minor digestive complaints that don't resolve themselves just by following the ONE BOWL concept.

Once you have expanded your attention into these areas of your life, you will see that the path of health and self-knowledge continues further still. You can begin to apply your tools of understanding and exploration to other parts of your body. There are two books I know which are new and excellent for this work. Both are very positive in their approach to body health and both are fairly comprehensive.

Getting Clear, Body Work For Women, by Anne Kent Rush can be used by men as well. It will show you how to explore your self and your relationships to others through exercises and by examining the many social roles you play. I have learned a great deal from it. The book has a food section devoted to the Pearsons' work, which makes it perfect as a guide to moving from your diet into the rest of your body life.

The Well Body Book, by Mike Samuels, M.D. and Hal Bennett is the most useful medical book I have ever seen. It shows you how to begin to diagnose and treat common illnesses and how to understand your body's natural healing processes. A large section on preventive medicine seems to fit right into my personal body exploration space.

Persons who carry their self-understanding this far are reaching toward the frontiers in this work. Preventive medicine is a rediscovered, expanding field devoted to physical and psychic self-exploration. I have mentioned these books because they can be stepping stones along your path. Most people I know who begin to understand and make changes in their diet want to go beyond this original goal. You can begin by wanting to lose a few pounds and end up transforming your basic ways of being in the world.

PEACE OF MIND

I began this quest by trying to lose twenty pounds. The time I spent just sitting, taking a bite of food every few minutes, listening to the food sensations inside me, led to several unexpected paths. For one, it led me to write this book. For another it led me into a space in which I am much more content with myself. This space is a direct result of wanting to focus on the food energy inside, but it has brought another world into view. ONE BOWL has carried me into a personal way of being that is more peaceful, that allows me to detach myself from my cares and to experience myself as a whole body, a living connected being without name or desire. This is a space in which I do not know myself by thinking and do not talk to myself with words. It is a silent space, a space of pure sensation. Within it I am a biological organism; I become my body. Body sensations are my language. I live life slowly, at what I imagine to be a biochemical rate of speed. I feel immensely calm and secure. I value this space in my life enough to try to enter it at least once a day.

Down through history people have discovered this kind of space for themselves and have called it by many names — prayer, meditation and being at one are a few of them. You can use the knowledge you have learned in ONE BOWL to begin to open yourself to this personal place too.

I get into this special space the same way I listen to food messages, except that now I listen for messages anywhere in my entire body, but not, of course, when I'm eating. I just close my eyes and listen for whatever is going on. I focus my attention first on the sensations of

> the pulsation of my heartbeat
>
> the rhythm of my breathing

and I try to relax any tensed muscles I feel. My breathing slows down; it falls lower into my abdomen. I just let it go. After a few moments of this I pay attention to sensations of

> falling
>
> tingling
>
> changes in weight, pressure, temperature
>
> emptiness

and soon it is just as though a door closed, shutting out the world. I am internally quiet, sometimes floating, at peace.

At first these feelings made me uneasy because they were quite unfamiliar. When I tried to evaluate them or interpret them I had difficulty keeping them in focus. Then, one day, I realized *that all these sensations, even the strangest ones, were me.* After that I found it easier to explore them. Now I am learning how to travel around among the sensations in my body and throughout its many parts. The more I follow this path, the more I secure for myself an inner sanctuary against the storm of my desires and ambitions. This brings me peace.

If you are a person who enjoys being quiet with yourself, you may enjoy this space. Any time you feel tense or hyperactive, you can find relaxation and well-being here. A good philosophical work that will bring you to this same conclusion from the tradition of Christian Theology is Soren Kierkegaard's *Purity of Heart is to Will One Thing.*

CREATING YOURSELF

I developed this diet path by using my common sense and because I believe that the feelings I feel inside me are real and are important to my well-being. I also believe that my body has the ability to choose how to be healthy, and *will always act,* in any situation, *in the most healthy way it can.*

As I experience the ONE BOWL concept each day my self-confidence grows. Good feelings about the role of food in my life help me rely more on my own power to care for myself.

These beliefs rest firmly on my experiences; they are reaffirmed and renewed continually in my daily life.

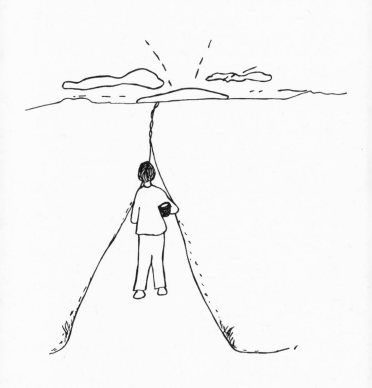